ISBN: 9781070616032

25-DAY
EASY DIET

1200 Calorie

Gail Johnson, M.S.

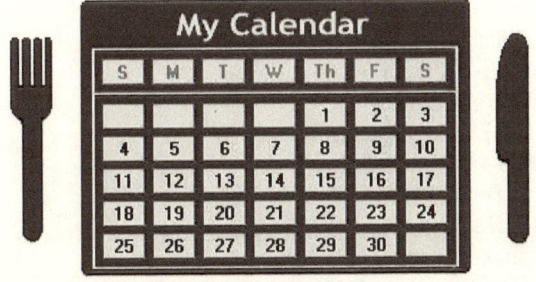

NoPaperPress™

Note: The no-cooking portions of this book rely, to a large extent, on off-the-shelf foods. At publication, these foods were widely available in most super-markets. But food products come and go. So if there is a frozen entrée or soup selection that is out of stock, or that's been discontinued, or perhaps you don't like, or that you forgot to pick up while shopping, please substitute another food that has **approximately** the same caloric value and nutritional content. In this regard, many dieters have found the foods listed in the Appendices at the end of this book to be helpful.

CONTENTS

Expected Weight Loss

Weight loss occurs when your food energy intake is less than the total energy you expend. This difference in calories is referred to as your calorie deficit. How much weight you lose depends on the magnitude of your calorie deficit. Physiologists know that to lose one pound requires a deficit of approximately 3500 Calories. Therefore, if a person's total calorie deficit over time is known, their weight loss over time can be calculated.

On the *25-Day Easy Diet – 1200 Calorie Edition*, **most women lose 9 to 14 lbs.** Smaller women, older women and less active women lose a bit less and larger women, younger women and more active women often lose much more.

On the *25-Day Easy Diet – 1200 Calorie Edition*, **most men lose 18 to 23 lbs**. Smaller men, older men and less active men will lose a tad less and larger men, younger men and more active men frequently lose much more.

Exactly how much weight you will lose depends on how much you weigh, your age and your activity level. For the full story see *Weight Control - U.S. Edition* by Vincent W. Antonetti, Ph.D., a book published by NoPaperPress.

Medical Checkup

Everyone should at the very least have a medical checkup before starting a weight loss diet. Why? You need to make sure your health will allow you to lower your caloric intake and increase your physical activity. The checkup may be as simple as a visit to a physician who is familiar with your medical history, or it may be a thorough physical exam. The physician conducting the medical exam should be made aware of and should approve the specific weight loss diet you're planning.

The Key to Healthy Eating

No single food can supply all the nutrients you need in the amounts you need. The most important factors in nutrition are variety, variety, variety! **Variety is the key to a nutritious diet.** As a means of setting strategies for food selection, the U.S. Department of Health and Human Services and the Department of Agriculture issue Dietary Guidelines every five years. The latest Dietary Guidelines describe a healthy diet as one that:

- Emphasizes fruits, vegetables, whole grains, and fat-free or low-fat milk products.
- Includes fish, poultry, lean meats, beans and nuts.
- Is low in saturated fats, trans fats, cholesterol, salt (sodium) and added sugars.

The guidelines encourage adults to consume a variety of nutrient-dense foods and beverages within their caloric needs. The afore mentioned U.S. government agency recommends how much should be eaten from each of the basic food groups (i.e., from the fruit group, vegetable group, grains group, meat and beans group, milk group, and oils group) – whether you are trying to lose weight or maintain your weight. All this information and more can be found in my book *Eat Smart - U.S. Edition* published by NoPaperPress.

Even though most adults can get all the vitamins and minerals they need by merely consuming a variety of nutritious foods (from the all the different groups), many physicians recommend a daily multi-vitamin/mineral supplement – just in case you don't eat the way you should.

Large Green Salad: One of the dinner mainstays of the *25-Day Easy Diet* is a "Large Green Salad." To prepare your "Large Green Salad" start with a bowl with a volume of at least 16 ounces, or 2 cups. First add about 1 cup of either green leaf lettuce, Romaine lettuce or a mesclun mix. Then add, as desired, half cup of green veggies such as broccoli, celery, cucumber, peppers, spinach, or watercress. This vegetable combination will, on average, total about 35 Calories. You will be eating a "Large Green Salad" just about every day at dinnertime. Remember that variety is the key to a nutritious diet. So be sure to vary the ingredients of the salad.

Top your "Large Green Salad" with 1½ tablespoons of any light salad dressing available at your local supermarket that contains no more than 25 Calories per tablespoon. Some of our favorite light salad dressings are:
  - **Ken's Steakhouse Fat Free Raspberry Pecan**
  - **Kraft Light Done Right House Italian**
  - **Wishbone Just 2 Good Honey Dijon**
  - **Newman's Lighten Up! Balsamic Vinaigrette**

Your "Large Green Salad" with salad dressing will cost you roughly 70 Calories but will be packed with lots of health-giving vitamins, minerals and fiber.

About Bread: First understand that bread, more specifically whole-grain breads, are good sources of complex carbohydrates and dietary fiber, as well as several B vitamins (thiamin, riboflavin, niacin, and foliate), vitamin E, and minerals (iron, magnesium and selenium). In recent years, however, sliced bread loaves have gotten larger, as have the bread slices inside these loaves. Just a few years ago the standard slice of bread contained about 65 to 70 Calories – now most are 100 plus Calories.

  The *25-Day Easy Diet* requires whole-grain bread at 65 to 70 Calories per slice. Quite a few bakers sell thin sliced or "light" sliced bread. The difficult part is finding a whole grain thin sliced or "light" bread (with about 70 Calories per slice). Whatever the brand, make sure the first word in the Ingredients List is "whole." "Pepperidge Farm Small Slice 100% Whole Wheat" is a good choice. It's whole grain, has 70 Calories per slice and it tastes good too.

Exchanging Foods

If there is a food listed in the *25-Day Easy Diet* that you don't like, or perhaps that you forgot to pick up while shopping, you probably can exchange or substitute another food in its place – a technique used by dieticians. Exchanging a food listed in a diet for another food with approximately equal caloric value and nutritional content is the foundation of a successful long-term diet. Substitution possibilities are almost endless but have to be done carefully.

  The easiest substitutions are those within the same food group, such as exchanging one vegetable variety for another, or a glass of milk for a cup of yogurt. More sophisticated exchanges cross food groups, for instance replacing 3½ ounces of turkey with a tablespoon of peanut butter spread on a piece of whole wheat bread. Both foods are complete protein and both contain about 175 Calories.

  Refer to the calorie table in **Appendix A** on page 62. With some understanding and experience, you can use this table to assist you make a substitution for a food listed in the *25-Day Easy Diet* with an equal calorie food from the same food group.

Breakfast: You may substitute any cereal for any other wholesome cereal. For example, if you're not crazy about having Shredded Wheat for breakfast on Day 6, substitute Wheat Chex or Cheerios, etc. If you don't like the soft-boiled egg called for on Day 9, make yourself a scrambled egg instead. And if Cantaloupe is on the menu but is not in season, replace the cantaloupe with a half cup of orange juice.

Snacks: Again, where yogurt is specified you may substitute an 8-ounce glass of skim milk, but to maintain a nutritionally balanced diet keep this snack a dairy selection. Similarly, when fruit is on the agenda, you may select another type of fruit but do not stray from the fruit group. Nuts and popcorn can be interchanged at will. (Incidentally, you should buy a hot-air popper. They make great popcorn – which is high in fiber and makes a tasty and nutritious snack.)

Two Nights Off

Everyone deserves a break from the grind of preparing dinner after coming home from work. So the *25-Day Easy Diet* gives you two days off per week! Notice that one night a week the meal plan calls for a frozen dinner and on a second night during the week you're encouraged to eat out. There are, however, some rules and caveats involved and these are covered in the next two sections.

Frozen Dinner Rules

In general, a frozen dinner should not be a meal in itself. Make sure you add a salad, fruit, bread etc. The frozen dinner you choose should come with at least one cup of cooked vegetables. If your frozen dinner doesn't measure up, add your own frozen, fresh or canned vegetables. And look for dinners with no more than 800 mg of sodium. In addition, make sure the dinner you choose has no more than 30 percent of the daily value for total fat.

And on the days when a frozen dinner is specified, you will also be given a calorie goal for the frozen dinner. For example, Day 5 calls for frozen fish dinner with a maximum allowable 300 Calories. If you choose a frozen fish dinner that contains less than 300 Calories, you may spend the unused calories any way you wish.

Moreover, on those nights when you just don't have the energy or time to cook, you can always substitute a frozen dinner for the entree listed in the meal plan. For example, Day 1 calls for Baked Cod dinner. The total allowable calorie count for dinner is 415. In place of the cod, any combination of a frozen fish dinner and side dishes (salads, etc) with a total calorie count close to 415 would be an acceptable, albeit not as tasty an alternative.

Eating Out Strategies

You may eat out once a week. When you're on a diet, however, eating in a restaurant can be a challenge, because most restaurant portions are huge, and can easily total more than 1000 Calories.

On the *25-Day Easy Diet*, a dinner type (i.e., fish, chicken, etc) and a calorie target is specified. For example Day 7 of the diet specifies a chicken dinner and allows you 580 Calories.

First, you need to choose a restaurant where you have a fighting chance to achieve your calorie goal. Next, order simple, such as broiled fish with steamed vegetables and brown rice. Tell the waiter you want no sauce, no gravy, nothing added. Then, knowing your calorie objective, and that most fish and chicken are about 50 Calories per ounce, most steamed vegetable servings average approximately 50 Calories per cup, and rice is about 100 Calories per ½ cup, decide how much to eat – and take the remainder home. If fresh fruit is not an option, pass on dessert and have the evening snack specified in the meal plan for that day.

Easy Diet Info

As mentioned previously, there are two diet plans in this book:
- 1200 Calorie daily menus start on page 10.
There is a detailed meal plan for each of the 25 days. Associated with each day is a "Recipe of the Day" and a "Diet Tip of the Day.
- Recipes of the Day start on page 36.
The 1,200 Calorie diet adheres to the United States Department of Agriculture recommendation that suggest a balanced diet should have approximately 50 percent of its calories from carbs, about 20 percent from protein sources and 30 percent or less from fat. (Note, the *25-Day Easy Diet* may not be appropriate for individuals with illnesses such as heart disease, diabetes, food allergies, etc. Again, please see your physician before starting this diet – or any diet.)

After you complete the 25th day on the diet, if you still want to lose more weight a good alternative is to repeat the diet by starting over at Day1.

Diet Notes

1) Coffee or tea may be decaf or regular. If desired, skim milk and a sugar substitute may be added to coffee or tea. Coffee may be regular or decaf. And soy or almond milk may be used instead of cow's milk. Fried eggs, scrambled eggs, or an omelet should be cooked in a pan coated with a non-stick cooking spray.

2) On bread, corn on the cob, baked potatoes, if desired, you may use a zero-calorie butter substitute spray.

3) Cereals should be whole grain and preferably with no added sugar. At the top of the list are Old-fashioned Oat Meal, Wheatena and Shredded Wheat. Among other reasonably healthy choices are Cheerios, Wheat Chex, Wheaties, some Kashi cereals and Farina. When blueberries are in season, you may add **blueberries instead of raisins** to your cereal. (Substitution ratio = 2 blueberries per raisin.)

4) Bread may be either plain or toasted whole grain, such as whole wheat, whole rye or pumpernickel. If desired, bread may be sprayed with a zero-calorie butter substitute.

5) Use only lean cuts of meat trimmed of all visible fat. Poultry should be limited to chicken or turkey breasts (white meat and skinless). **Turkey bacon** should contain no more than 35 Calories per slice.

6) When canned tuna or salmon is specified, use only fish packed in water.

7) An unlimited amount of green salad may be eaten, but the salad dressing should be as specified. (Incidentally, in the meal plans Evoo means extra virgin olive oil.)

8) Use freely as desired: clear unsweetened coffee, clear unsweetened tea, water, seltzer water and any diet soda.

9) Use freely as desired: clear soups without fat, bouillon, and seasonings such as mustard, cinnamon, dill, herbs, red and black pepper, curry, vinegar, lemon juice and sections, and dill and sour pickles.

10) On days when a leftover is specified for lunch. Eat about half as much as you ate for dinner a night or two before.

11) Any specified snack may be moved to any other part of the day, and/or combined with breakfast, lunch or dinner.

12) Take a daily multi-vitamin/mineral supplement. This is important when you're on a diet – as a kind of insurance policy.

1200-CALORIE DAILY MENUS

Day 1 – 1200 Calorie Meal Plan

BREAKFAST	Calories	Totals
Orange juice (½ cup)	50	
Wheaties (¾ cup) + ½ cup skim milk + ½ banana	190	
Coffee (See page 9)	10	250 Cal
SNACK		
Fresh fruit in season (apple, peach, etc)	70	70 Cal
LUNCH		
Soup (Appendix C - page 71)	110	
Turkey breast (1 oz) on 1 slice rye bread	105	
Pickle spear	0	
Lettuce & tomato slices	20	
Coffee or tea	10	245 Cal
SNACK		
One small cookie*	80	
Skim milk (4 oz)	40	120 Cal
DINNER		
Baked Herb-Crusted Cod (Day 1 Recipe - page 37)	230	
Spinach (½ cup) steamed with garlic & drizzled	100	
Asparagus (7 spear cooked & drained)	20	
Whole-grain Bread (page 6) (1 slice)	65	
Water	0	415 Cal
SNACK		
Fiber One Chocolate Fudge Brownie	90	
Coffee or tea	10	100 Cal
* Oatmeal, ginger snap, sugar, etc - check calories!		1200 Cal

Day 2 – 1200 Calorie Meal Plan

BREAKFAST	Calories	Totals
Fresh or frozen strawberries (½ cup)	25	
French toasted English Muffin (Day 2 Recipe - page 38)	270	
Light syrup (1 Tbsp)	30	
Coffee	10	335 Cal
SNACK		
Coffee or tea	10	10 Cal
LUNCH		
Salad (3 oz tuna, 1 tsp Evoo, onions & celery)	175	
Lettuce & tomato wedges	20	
Fresh fruit in season (apple, peach, etc)	70	
Diet soda or water	0	265 Cal
SNACK		
Yogurt (6 oz, nonfat, any flavor)*	90	
Coffee or tea	10	100 Cal
DINNER		
Broiled veal chop (4 oz lean)	200	
Corn on the cob (1 medium ear)	100	
Broccoli (½ cup steamed)	25	
Large green salad** w 1½ Tbsp low-cal dressing	70	
Water	0	395 Cal
** See page 5.		
SNACK		
Graham crackers (3 squares)	90	
Coffee or tea	10	100 Cal
* Such as Dannon Lite & Fit. Buy 32 oz container - use 6 oz		1205 Cal

Day 3 – 1200 Calorie Meal Plan

BREAKFAST	Calories	Totals
Grapefruit (½)	75	
Scrambled egg (page 9)	80	
Whole-grain toast (1 slice) (page 6)	65	
Coffee	10	230 Cal
SNACK		
Coffee or tea	10	10 Cal
LUNCH		
Open face sandwich (2 oz ham & 1 slice rye bread)	225	
Pickle spear	0	
Small bunch of grapes	65	
Diet soda or water	0	290 Cal
SNACK		
Yogurt (6 oz, nonfat, any flavor)	90	
Coffee or tea	10	100 Cal
DINNER		
Chicken w Peppers & Onions (Day 3 Recipe - page 39)	250	
Sautéed red peppers with onions	70	
Green beans (steamed) & mashed cauliflower	45	
Large green salad with 1½ Tbsp low-cal dressing	70	
Whole-grain bread (1 slice)	65	
Water	0	500 Cal
SNACK		
Fresh fruit in season (apple, plum, etc)	70	70 Cal
		1200 Cal

Day 4 – 1200 Calorie Meal Plan

BREAKFAST	Calories	Totals
Grapefruit (½)	75	
Cheerios (1 cup) + ½ cup skim milk + about 15 raisins*	190	
Coffee	10	275 Cal
SNACK		
Coffee or tea	10	10 Cal
LUNCH		
Subway 6" (Roast Beef, Cheese + veggies)*	245	
Large tossed salad with 1½ Tbsp low-cal dressing	70	
Hot or iced tea	10	325 Cal
* On 6" half wheat roll.		
SNACK		
Fresh fruit in season (peach, plum, etc)	70	
Coffee or tea	10	80 Cal
DINNER		
Meat Loaf (Day 4 Recipe - page 40)	290	
One-half acorn squash (baked with ½ tsp maple	90	
Spinach (½ cup steamed & drizzled with 1 tsp	70	
Romaine lettuce, tomato slices & 1 Tbsp low-cal	45	
Hot or iced tea	10	505 Cal
SNACK		
Coffee or tea	10	10 Cal
* See page 9 re substituting blueberries for raisins.		1200 Cal

Day 5 – 1200 Calorie Meal Plan

BREAKFAST	Calories	Totals
Cantaloupe (½ medium)	50	
Fried egg	80	
Toasted raisin bread (1 slice)	75	
Coffee	10	215 Cal
SNACK		
Coffee or tea	10	10 Cal
LUNCH		
Soup (Appendix C - page 72)	130	
Small whole-grain roll	80	
Lettuce and sliced tomato + 1 Tbsp low-cal	45	
Canned pineapple (½ cup, no-sugar-added juice)	40	
Hot or iced tea	10	305 Cal
SNACK		
Yogurt (6 oz, nonfat, any flavor)	90	
Coffee or tea	10	100 Cal
DINNER		
Frozen fish dinner (Day 5 Recipe - page 41)	340	
Large green salad with 1½ Tbsp low-cal dressing	70	
Water	0	410 Cal
SNACK		
Graham crackers (3 squares)	90	
Skim milk (6 oz)	70	150 Cal
		1200 Cal

Day 6 – 1200 Calorie Meal Plan

BREAKFAST	Calories	Totals
Tomato juice (½ cup)	20	
Shredded Wheat (1 cup) + ½ cup skim milk + ½ banana	265	
Coffee	10	295 Cal
SNACK		
Coffee or tea	10	10 Cal
LUNCH		
Leftover meat loaf (½ Day 4 serving size) w ketchup	155	
Small whole-grain roll	80	
Lettuce	0	
Fresh or frozen berries (½ cup)	50	
Hot or iced tea	10	295 Cal
SNACK		
Yogurt (6 oz, nonfat, any flavor)	90	
Coffee or tea	10	100 Cal
DINNER		
Pizza (Day 6 Recipe - page 42)	350	
Large green salad with 1½ Tbsp low-cal dressing	70	
Fresh fruit in season (pear, plum, etc)	70	
Water	0	490 Cal
SNACK		
Coffee or tea	10	10 Cal
		1200 Cal

Day 7 – 1200 Calorie Meal Plan

BREAKFAST	Calories	Totals
Cantaloupe (½ medium)	50	
Oatmeal (½ cup dry) + ½ cup skim milk + about 15 raisins	220	
Coffee	10	280 Cal
SNACK		
Coffee or tea	10	10 Cal
LUNCH		
Grilled cheese sandwich (2 slices 2% cheese)	230	
Lettuce and sliced tomato	20	
Pickle spear	0	
Water	0	250 Cal
SNACK		
Carrot sticks + ¼ cup low-fat cottage cheese & chives	60	
Coffee or tea	10	70 Cal
DINNER		
Eat Out – Chicken dinner (Day 7 Recipe - page 43)		
Max allowable calories	580	580 Cal
SNACK		
Coffee or tea	10	10 Cal
		1200 Cal

Day 8 – 1200 Calorie Meal Plan

BREAKFAST	Calories	Totals
Cantaloupe (½ medium)	50	
Wheaties (¾ cup) + ½ cup skim milk + ½ banana	190	
Coffee	10	250 Cal
SNACK		
Coffee or tea	10	10 Cal
LUNCH		
Subway 6" (Turkey Breast, Cheese + veggies)	230	
Canned pineapple (½ cup, no-sugar-added juice)	40	
Hot or iced tea	10	280 Cal
SNACK		
Coffee or tea	10	10 Cal
DINNER		
Baked salmon with salsa (Day 8 Recipe - page 44)	215	
Summer squash, zucchini and tomatoes	60	
Brown rice (½ cup)	100	
Large green salad with 1½ Tbsp low-cal dressing	70	
Fresh fruit in season (apple, plum, etc)	70	
Water with lemon wedge	15	530 Cal
SNACK		
Popcorn Mini Bag*	110	
Coffee or tea	10	120 Cal
* Such as Orville Redenbacher's Smart Pop		1200 Cal

Day 9 – 1200 Calorie Meal Plan

BREAKFAST	Calories	Totals
Orange juice (½ cup)	50	
Soft-boiled egg	80	
Whole-grain toast (1 slice)	65	
Coffee	10	205 Cal
SNACK		
Coffee or tea	10	10 Cal
LUNCH		
Salad (3 oz tuna, 1 tsp Evoo, onions & celery)	175	
Lettuce & tomato wedges	20	
Rye bread (1 slice)	65	
Fresh fruit in season (pear, peach, etc)	70	
Diet soda or water	0	330 Cal
SNACK		
Yogurt (6 oz, nonfat, any flavor)	90	90 Cal
DINNER		
Veggie burger – (1 patty) (Day 9 Recipe - page 45)	100	
Low-fat cheddar cheese (1 thin slice)	50	
Seeded hamburger roll + Beets (3 small)	140	
Large green salad with 1½ Tbsp low-cal dressing	70	
Fresh fruit in season (apple, peach, etc)	70	
Water	0	475 Cal
SNACK		
One small cookie	80	
Coffee or tea	10	90 Cal
		1200 Cal

Day 10 – 1200 Calorie Meal Plan

BREAKFAST	Calories	Totals
Orange juice (½ cup)	50	
Wild blueberry pancakes (Day 10 Recipe - page 46)	190	
Light syrup (1½ Tbsp)	45	
Coffee	10	295 Cal
SNACK		
Coffee or tea	10	10 Cal
LUNCH		
Peanut butter (2 Tbsp) on 2 slices whole-grain bread	330	
Skim milk (6 oz)	70	
Fresh fruit in season (apple, plum, etc)	70	470 Cal
SNACK		
Coffee or tea	10	10 Cal
DINNER		
Broiled pork chop (about ½" thick & trimmed of fat)	260	
Green peas (½ cup)	55	
Tomato & cucumber salad with 2 Tbsp low-cal	70	
Water with lemon section	15	400 Cal
SNACK		
Coffee or tea	10	10 Cal
		1195 Cal

Day 11 – 1200 Calorie Meal Plan

BREAKFAST	Calories	Totals
Fresh sliced orange	75	
Cheerios (1 cup) + ½ cup skim milk + about 15 raisins	190	
Coffee	10	275 Cal
SNACK		
Fresh fruit in season (apple, plum, etc)	70	
Coffee or tea	10	80 Cal
LUNCH		
Cottage cheese (1 cup low fat)	180	
Large green salad with 1½ Tbsp low-cal dressing	70	
Small whole-grain roll	80	
Hot or iced tea	10	340 Cal
SNACK		
Handful unsalted mixed nuts	100	100 Cal
DINNER		
Grilled chicken sausage (2 links about 2½ oz per link)	180	
Artichoke-bean salad (Day 11 Recipe - page 47)	190	
Green beans - steamed	25	
Water	0	395 Cal
SNACK		
Coffee or tea	10	10 Cal
		1200 Cal

Day 12 – 1200 Calorie Meal Plan

BREAKFAST	Calories	Totals
Grapefruit (½)	75	
Scrambled egg	80	
Whole-grain toast (1 slice)	65	
Coffee	10	230 Cal
SNACK		
Coffee or tea	10	10 Cal
LUNCH		
Southwest-Style Taco*	270	
Diet soda or water	0	270 Cal
* Hot Pockets (wrap)		
SNACK		
Yogurt (6 oz, nonfat, any flavor)	90	90 Cal
DINNER		
Eat Out – Fish dinner (Day 12 Recipe - page 48)		
Max allowable calories	595	595 Cal
SNACK		
Coffee or tea	10	10 Cal
		1205 Cal

Day 13 – 1200 Calorie Meal Plan

BREAKFAST	Calories	Totals
Orange juice (½ cup)	50	
Shredded Wheat (1 cup) + ½ cup skim milk + ½ banana	260	
Coffee	10	320 Cal
SNACK		
Coffee or tea	10	10 Cal
LUNCH		
Turkey frank (2 oz) with mustard & relish	150	
Hot dog bun	130	
Gelatin dessert (unsweetened)	10	
Hot or iced tea	10	300 Cal
SNACK		
Coffee or tea	10	10 Cal
DINNER		
Pasta w Marinara sauce (Day 13 Recipe - page 49)	225	
Large green salad with 1½ Tbsp low-cal dressing	70	
Fresh fruit in season (pear, plum, etc)	70	
Italian or French bread (1 slice)	80	
Water with lemon section	15	460 Cal
SNACK		
Fiber One Chocolate Fudge Brownie	90	
Coffee or tea	10	100 Cal
		1200 Cal

Day 14 – 1200 Calorie Meal Plan

BREAKFAST	Calories	Totals
Cantaloupe (½ medium)	50	
Oatena cereal mix (Day 14 Recipe - page 50)	310	
Coffee	10	370 Cal
SNACK		
Coffee or tea	10	10 Cal
LUNCH		
Grilled Swiss cheese sandwich (2 oz low-fat cheese)	240	
Pickle spear	0	
Hot or iced tea	10	250 Cal
SNACK		
Fresh fruit in season (apple, plum, etc)	70	
Coffee or tea	10	80 Cal
DINNER		
Frozen chicken dinner (Day 14b Recipe - page 51)	300	
Large green salad with 1½ Tbsp low-cal dressing	70	
Water with lemon wedge	15	385 Cal
SNACK		
Yogurt (6 oz, nonfat, any flavor)	90	
Coffee or tea	10	100 Cal
		1195 Cal

Day 15 – 1200 Calorie Meal Plan

BREAKFAST	Calories	Totals
Fresh or frozen strawberries (1 cup)	50	
French toast (made with 2 slices whole-grain	250	
Light syrup (1 Tbsp)	30	
Coffee	10	340 Cal
SNACK		
Coffee or tea	10	10 Cal
LUNCH		
Salad (3 oz tuna, 1 tsp Evoo, onions & celery)	175	
Lettuce & tomato wedges	20	
Rye bread (1 slice)	65	
Coffee or tea	10	270 Cal
SNACK		
Yogurt (6 oz, nonfat, any flavor)	90	
Coffee or tea	10	100 Cal
DINNER		
London broil (Day 15 Recipe - page 52)	320	
Brown rice (½ cup)	100	
Broccoli (1 cup steamed)	50	
Water	0	470 Cal
SNACK		
Coffee or tea	10	10 Cal
		1200 Cal

Day 16 – 1200 Calorie Meal Plan

BREAKFAST	Calories	Totals
Orange juice (½ cup)	50	
Wheat Chex (¾ cup) + ½ cup skim milk + ½ banana	250	
Coffee	10	310 Cal
SNACK		
Coffee or tea	10	10 Cal
LUNCH		
Subway 6" (Roast Beef, Cheese + veggies)	245	
Hot or iced tea	10	255 Cal
SNACK		
Fresh fruit in season (apple, peach, etc)	70	70 Cal
DINNER		
Baked red snapper (Day 16 Recipe - page 53)	215	
Wild rice mix	160	
Green beans & tomato	75	
Water with lemon section	15	465 Cal
SNACK		
Yogurt (6 oz, nonfat, any flavor)	90	90 Cal
		1200 Cal

Day 17 – 1200 Calorie Meal Plan

BREAKFAST	Calories	Totals
Cantaloupe (½ medium)	50	
Fried egg	80	
Turkey bacon (1 slice) (page 9)	35	
Toasted raisin bread (1 slice)	75	
Coffee	10	250 Cal
SNACK		
Coffee or tea	10	10 Cal
LUNCH		
Soup (Appendix C - page 72)	160	
Lettuce & tomato sandwich (Tbsp light mayo)	170	
Cucumber slices and carrot & celery sticks	15	
Hot or iced tea	10	355 Cal
SNACK		
Yogurt (6 oz, nonfat, any flavor)	90	
Coffee or tea	10	100 Cal
DINNER		
Cajun chicken salad (Day 17 Recipe - page 54)	330	
Whole-grain bread (1 slice)	65	
Fresh fruit in season (pear, plum, etc)	70	
Hot or iced tea	10	475 Cal
SNACK		
Coffee or tea	10	10 Cal
		1200 Cal

Day 18 – 1200 Calorie Meal Plan

BREAKFAST	Calories	Totals
Grapefruit (½)	75	
Cheerios (1 cup) + ½ cup skim milk + about 15 raisins	190	
Coffee	10	275 Cal
SNACK		
Coffee or tea	10	80 Cal
LUNCH		
Cottage cheese (1 cup low fat)	180	
Large green salad with 1½ Tbsp low-cal dressing	70	
Hot or iced tea	10	260 Cal
SNACK		
Handful unsalted mixed nuts	100	
Coffee or tea	10	110 Cal
DINNER		
Grilled swordfish (Day 18 Recipe - page 55)	250	
Grilled potatoes	100	
Grilled cherry tomatoes	45	
Spinach (½ cup) steamed with garlic & drizzled	50	
Water with lemon section	15	460 Cal
SNACK		
Coffee or tea	10	10 Cal
		1195 Cal

Day 19 – 1200 Calorie Meal Plan

BREAKFAST	Calories	Totals
Grapefruit (½)	75	
Scrambled egg	80	
Whole-grain toast (1 slice)	65	
Coffee	10	230 Cal
SNACK		
Coffee or tea	10	10 Cal
LUNCH		
Soup (Appendix C - page 72)	190	
Turkey (1 oz) on 1 slice rye bread (½ sandwich)	115	
Diet soda or water	0	305 Cal
SNACK		
Coffee or tea	10	10 Cal
DINNER		
Eat Out – Chinese food (Day 19 Recipe - page 56)		
Max allowable calories	640	640 Cal
SNACK		
Coffee or tea	10	10 Cal
		1205 Cal

Day 20 – 1200 Calorie Meal Plan

BREAKFAST	Calories	Totals
Tomato juice (½ cup)	20	
Shredded Wheat (1 cup) + ½ cup skim milk + ½ banana	260	
Coffee	10	290 Cal
SNACK		
Coffee or tea	10	10 Cal
LUNCH		
Left over Chinese food (Day 19 Recipe - page 56)	260	
Hot or iced tea	10	270 Cal
SNACK		
Yogurt (6 oz, nonfat, any flavor)	90	
Coffee or tea	10	100 Cal
DINNER		
Spaghetti alla Puttanesca (Day 20 Recipe - page 57)	345	
Large green salad with 1½ Tbsp low-cal dressing	70	
Water with lemon section	15	430 Cal
SNACK		
Coffee or tea	10	10 Cal
		1200 Cal

Day 21 – 1200 Calorie Meal Plan

BREAKFAST	Calories	Totals
Cantaloupe (½ medium)	50	
Oatmeal (½ cup dry) + ½ cup skim milk + about 15 raisins	220	
Coffee	10	**280 Cal**
SNACK		
Coffee or tea	10	**10 Cal**
LUNCH		
Turkey breast (2 oz) sandwich	235	
Lettuce & tomato with Tbsp light mayo	35	
Pickle spear	0	
Fresh fruit in season (apple, plum, etc)	70	
Hot or iced tea	10	**350 Cal**
SNACK		
Yogurt (6 oz, nonfat, any flavor)	90	
Coffee or tea	10	**100 Cal**
DINNER		
Frozen meat dinner (Day 21 Recipe - page 58)	300	
Large green salad with 1½ Tbsp low-cal dressing	70	
Whole-grain bread (1 slice)	65	
Water with lemon section	15	**450 Cal**
SNACK		
Coffee or tea	10	**10 Cal**
		1200 Cal

Day 22 – 1200 Calorie Meal Plan

BREAKFAST	Calories	Totals
Fresh or frozen strawberries (1 cup)	25	
French toasted English Muffin (Day 2 Recipe - page 38)	270	
Light syrup (1 Tbsp)	30	
Coffee	10	335 Cal
SNACK		
Coffee or tea	10	10 Cal
LUNCH		
Soup (Appendix C - page 72)	140	
BLT sandwich (2 slices turkey bacon, 1 Tbsp light	235	
Pickle spear	0	
Hot or iced tea	10	385 Cal
SNACK		
Coffee or tea	10	10 Cal
DINNER		
Shrimp & spinach salad (Day 22 Recipe - page 59)	310	
Whole-grain bread (1 slice)	65	
Large green salad with 1½ Tbsp low-cal dressing	70	
Water	0	445 Cal
SNACK		
Coffee or tea	10	10 Cal
		1195 Cal

Day 23 – 1200 Calorie Meal Plan

BREAKFAST	Calories	Totals
Cantaloupe (½ medium)	50	
Wheaties (¾ cup) + ½ cup skim milk + ½ banana	190	
Whole-grain toast (1 slice)	65	
Coffee	10	315 Cal
SNACK		
Coffee or tea	10	10 Cal
LUNCH		
Ham (2 oz) with mustard on 2 slices rye bread	290	
Pickle spear	0	
Lettuce & tomato wedges	20	
Hot or iced tea	10	320 Cal
SNACK		
Handful unsalted mixed nuts	100	
Coffee or tea	10	110 Cal
DINNER		
Beans & greens salad (Day 23 Recipe - page 60)	260	
Baked potato (medium)	100	
Fresh fruit in season (apple, peach, etc)	70	
Water	0	430 Cal
SNACK		
Coffee or tea	10	10 Cal
		1195 Cal

Day 24 – 1200 Calorie Meal Plan

BREAKFAST	Calories	Totals
Fresh orange sliced	75	
Soft-boiled egg	80	
Whole-grain toast (1 slice)	65	
Coffee	10	230 Cal
SNACK		
Yogurt (6 oz, nonfat, any flavor)	90	
Coffee or tea	10	100 Cal
LUNCH		
Salad – 3 oz salmon, 1 tsp Evoo, onions & celery	200	
Lettuce & tomato wedges	20	
Rye bread (1 slice)	65	
Coffee or tea	10	295 Cal
SNACK		
Fresh fruit in season (peach, plum, etc)	70	
Coffee or tea	10	80 Cal
DINNER		
Chicken breast – broiled (5 oz)	250	
Four bean plus salad (½ cup) (Day 24 Recipe-p.61)	135	
Large green salad with 1½ Tbsp low-cal dressing	70	
Gelatin dessert (unsweetened)	10	
Water with lemon wedge	15	480 Cal
SNACK		
Coffee or tea	10	10 Cal
		1195 Cal

Day 25 – 1200 Calorie Meal Plan

BREAKFAST	Calories	Totals
Cantaloupe (½ medium)	50	
Fried egg	80	
Toasted whole-grain bread (1 slice)	65	
Coffee	10	205 Cal
SNACK		
Yogurt (6 oz, nonfat, any flavor)	90	
Coffee or tea	10	100 Cal
LUNCH		
Soup (Appendix C - page 72)	200	
Hard whole-grain roll (medium)	80	
Lettuce & tomato slices	20	
Hot or iced tea	10	310 Cal
SNACK		
Fresh fruit in season (apple, plum, etc)	70	
Coffee or tea	10	80 Cal
DINNER		
Grilled scallops (Day 25 Recipe - page 62)	210	
Grilled polenta (Day 25 Recipe)	125	
Mushroom-steamed green beans-red onion (Day 25)	45	
Grilled asparagus	10	
Water	0	390 Cal
SNACK		
Popcorn Mini Bag	110	
Coffee or tea	10	120 Cal
		1205 Cal

RECIPES & DIET TIPS

Day 1 Recipe

Baked Herb-Crusted Cod

4 cod fish fillets (4 to 5 ounces each)
2 tablespoons flour
2 tablespoons cornmeal
2 tablespoons minced fresh herbs
2 teaspoons lemon juice

Sprinkle cod with lemon juice. Mix flour, cornmeal and herbs and dust the cod with the cornmeal-herb mixture. Bake in oven at 375 ºF for 10 minutes. Add salt and black pepper to taste.

Serves 4. One serving is about 230 Calories (for cod only).

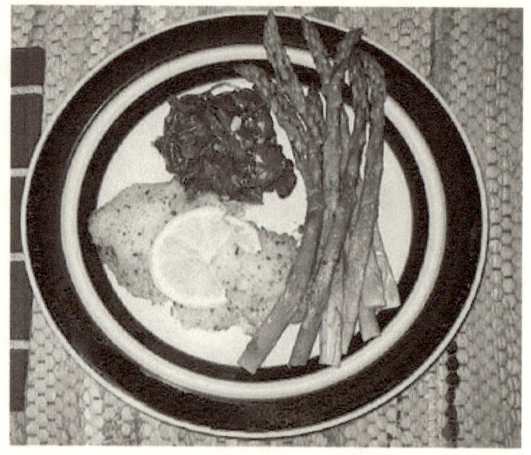

Diet Tip of the Day:. A **reducing diet is best supervised by a physician**. This is especially true when a great deal of weight needs to be lost, or if you have an ailment or a history of medical problems.

Day 2 Recipe
French-Toasted English Muffin

6 whole grain English muffins (light)
4 eggs
2 cups skim milk
2 teaspoons (tsp) vanilla
Dash of cinnamon

In a medium bowl, beat together eggs and skim milk. Add vanilla and cinnamon. Separate English muffins into halves and saturate slices in egg mixture. In a non-stick skillet coated with cooking spray, cook muffins until both sides are golden brown. Dust lightly with confectionary sugar. Serve hot or keep in an oven or warmer at 200 °F until ready to plate.

Serves 4. Three English muffin slices (1½ muffins) per serving. Serving is 270 Calories.

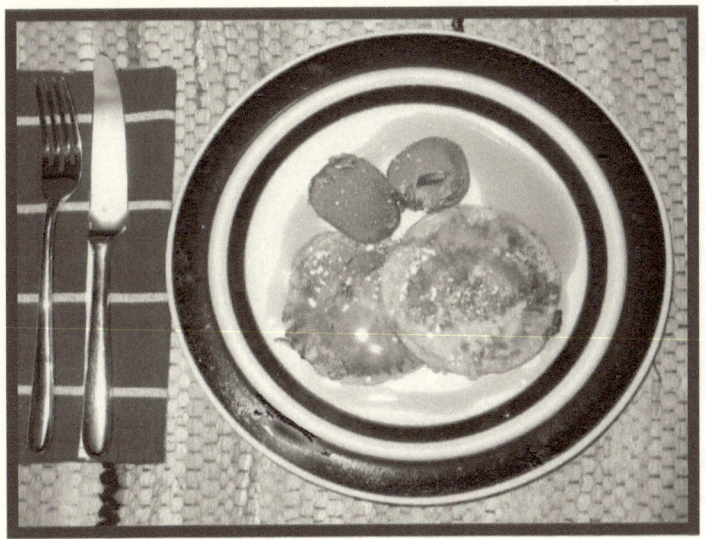

Diet Tip of the Day: "Eat Slowly" This is especially vital when you are trying to lose weight. If you are someone who eats fast, who finishes before everyone else at the table, you are not giving yourself a chance to feel full. While everyone else is still eating, you either sit there and pick, or you have seconds, taking in extra calories you could avoid if you would just slow down.

Day 3 Recipe
Chicken with Peppers & Onions

4 boneless & skinless chicken breasts (~ 5 oz each)

Coat the chicken breasts in a bottled barbeque sauce. Prepare medium-hot fire on well-oiled gas or charcoal grill . Place breasts on grill, turning them every 4 minutes, for 10 to 12 minutes, or until done. (To check if breasts are done, the meat should be moist and white with no sign of pink when you cut into breast.) Serve hot.

2 medium red peppers

1 medium onion

Place peppers and onions in pan with 2 Tbsp fat-free chicken stock. Sauté until stock is reduced. Spray pan lightly with non-stick cooking oil and sauté another 2 minutes. Salt and pepper to taste.

Serves 4. About 250 Calories per serving (for chicken only).

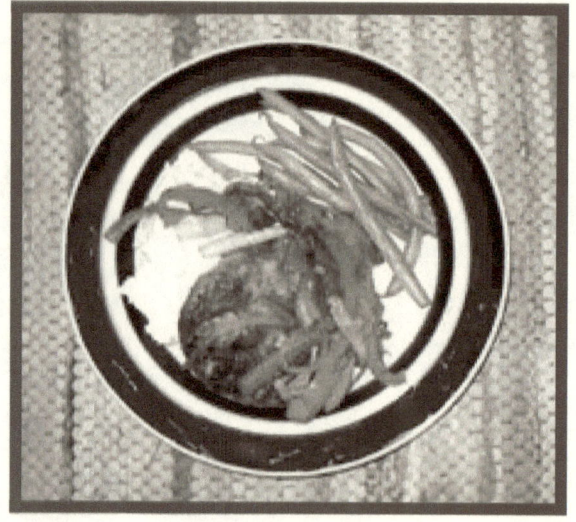

Diet Tip of the Day:. **A reducing diet is best supervised by a physician**. This is especially true when a great deal of weight needs to be lost, or if you have an ailment or a history of medical problems.

Day 4 Recipe
Meat Loaf

½ pound ground white meat turkey
½ pound ground beef (about 90% lean)
1 large egg
½ cup skim milk
¼ cup bread crumbs
¼ cup ketchup
¼ cup chopped carrots
¼ cup chopped onion

In a medium bowl, combine all ingredients. Add salt and pepper to taste.
Mix until blended and form into a loaf. Place loaf into oven preheated to
350 °F. Bake until an instant-read thermometer inserted in the center of
the loaf reads 160 °F. This should take about one hour.

Shown below is meat loaf, acorn squash baked with 1 tsp maple syrup
and steamed spinach drizzled with extra-virgin olive oil (Evoo).

Serves 5. Each serving of meat loaf is about 290 Calories (for meat loaf
only).

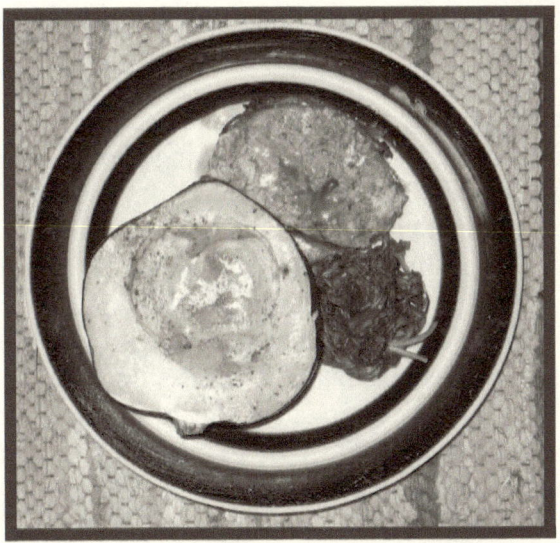

Diet Tip of the Day: Keep a daily food log to record everything you
eat. It really does work wonders.

Day 5 Recipe
Frozen-Fish Dinner
No recipe today. No cooking today. It's your day off! Some reasonably good frozen fish dinners are:

Seafood	Shrimp Alfredo	Lean Cuisine	~~230~~ 240
Seafood	Tuna Noodle Casserole	Smart Ones	~~250~~ 270
Seafood	Shrimp & Angel Hair Pasta	Lean Cuisine	~~280~~ 290
Seafood	Parmesan Crusted Fish	Lean Cuisine	~~290~~ 300
Seafood	Tortilla Crusted Fish	Lean Cuisine	~~300~~ 310

That's it. At this writing, there are just not that many frozen fish dinners for sale at supermarkets. If you choose any of the entrees, you will not use all of the **340 Calories allocated for this meal**. In this case, use the excess 100 or so calories anyway you wish. Splurge on extra dessert or save the calories for another day!

Please read the important **Frozen-Food Safety Warning** in **Appendix B, page 70.**

<u>Diet Tip of the Day:</u> **Buy a pedometer** and start walking. For the average person 2100 steps amounts to walking about one mile. A Harvard study has shown that 8000 to 10,000 step per day promote weight loss. And you're not obliged to walk continuously until you accrue all 10,000 steps. Rather, all steps throughout the day to wherever and whenever count toward your daily total. Because 10,000 steps a day may not be achievable by some people, particularly those who are elderly, sedentary, or who have chronic diseases, rather than insisting on a blanket 10,000 steps per day, your initial stepping goal should your baseline steps plus an increment of an additional 2500 steps. (Your baseline being the number of steps you take in an average day.)

Day 6 Recipe

Grandma's Pizza

The following is a pizza recipe used by my Italian grandmother. She was from a small mountain village located between Rome and Naples.

Pizza dough: To save time use prepared dough, preferably whole grain. Flour a large cutting board. <u>Divide one pound of prepared pizza dough into four parts</u>. Roll out each dough ball as thin as possible.

Tomato sauce: Sauté ½ small onion, chopped fine, in 1 tsp olive oil. Add two finely chopped garlic cloves, 1½ cups chopped plum tomatoes and ½ tsp chopped fresh oregano. Stir and cook about 5 minutes on a low flame.

Pizza preparation & cooking: On each pizza, spread evenly about ¼ cup of the tomato sauce. Add about ½ ounce of shredded part-skim mozzarella cheese, 1 tsp Parmesan cheese, 3 slices of a Portobello mushroom, some torn fresh basil, and drizzle with Evoo. Put pizzas on a pan and place in 475 °F oven for about 15 to 20 minutes, or until crust is crisp and cheese is just melting. (Freeze left over sauce for use on Day 13.)

<u>Serves 4</u>. Make four pizzas. Each pizza contains about 350 Calories.

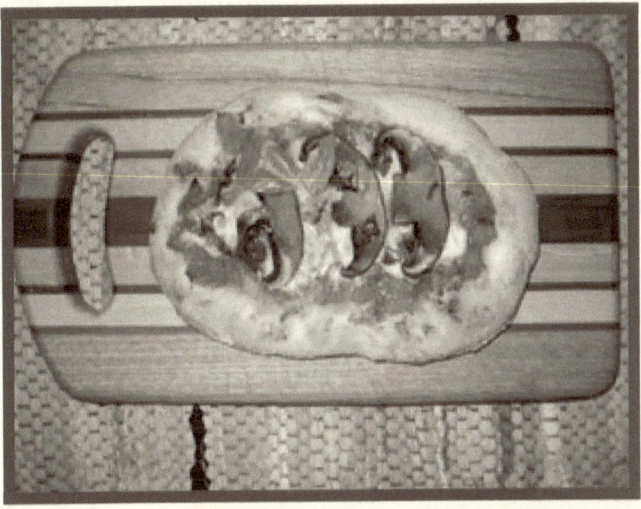

<u>Diet Tip of the Day:</u> For **life-long weight control** take a vigorous 30 to 60 minute walk everyday! That's right – everyday. Make exercise a nonflexible top priority part of your life. When it comes to exercise the key words are consistent, persistent, unyielding, dogged. Get the point?

Day 7 Recipe

Chicken Dinner - Out

No recipe today. No cooking today. Have a chicken dinner at your favorite restaurant, but make sure you choose a restaurant where you have a fighting chance to achieve your calorie goal. Your goal for dinner is a **maximum of 630 Calories**. This includes appetizer, soup, main course and dessert.

Tips for Eating Out: First, order simple, such as broiled chicken breast with steamed vegetables and brown rice. Tell the waiter you want no sauce, no gravy, nothing added. Then, knowing your calorie objective, and that chicken is about 50 Calories per ounce, most steamed vegetable servings average approximately 50 Calories per cup, and rice is about 100 Calories per ½ cup, decide how much to eat – and take the remainder home. If fresh fruit is not an option, pass on dessert and have the evening snack specified for that day in the diet.

In a restaurant, some nutritionists recommend you eat the low-calorie items on your plate first. Start with the salad, soup and veggies. By the time you get to the chicken and starches you will hopefully be full enough to be content with smaller portions of the higher-calorie choices.

Finally, some dieticians advise their dieting clients not to eat out. That's right. They believe eating at home is safer. But our thought is you have to eat out eventually so why not learn how while your resolve is high?

<u>Diet Tip of the Day:</u> When you're on a diet, eating in a restaurant can be a challenge, because most restaurant portions are huge, and can easily total more than 1,000 Calories. When eating in a restaurant decide how much to eat – and take the remainder home. A good general rule of thumb is to **eat half and bring the rest home**.

Day 8 Recipe

Baked Salmon with Salsa

This is a simple, straight-forward recipe. Again, the advantage of a simple recipe is there are no hidden calories.

4 5 oz salmon fillets
6 Tbsp bottled tomato-pepper salsa

Brown salmon fillets in non-stick pan and place in baking dish. Put fillets in an oven preheated to 350 °F for about 10 minutes. Plate the salmon. Stir prepared tomato-pepper salsa and spoon it over the salmon. **Serves 4**. One salmon fillet is about 215 Calories.

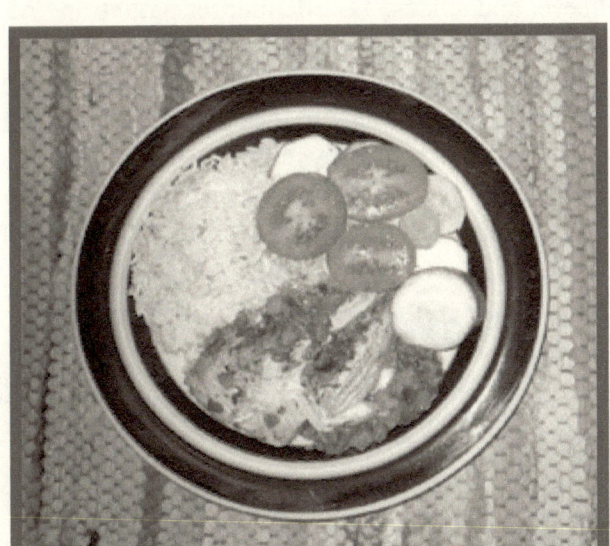

Diet Tip of the Day: **Have soup more often.** Most <u>non-cream-based</u> soups are filling and low-calorie.

Day 9 Recipe

Veggie Burger

Vegetable-based burgers can be purchased at your local supermarket. The patty of a veggie burger can be made from vegetables, soy, nuts, mushrooms, textured vegetable protein, dairy, or a combination of these foods.

Two popular veggie burgers are the Boca Burger and Gardenburger. The Boca Burger is made chiefly from soy protein and grain gluten. (Boca Burger patties are 2.5 oz each and range from 60 to 90 Calories.) The original Gardenburger is made from mushrooms, onions, brown rice, rolled oats, cheese, and spices. (Gardenburger patties are 2.5 oz each and about 100 Calories.)

To prepare, follow package directions. The version shown below has an added slice of low-fat cheddar cheese. The lettuce, tomato and ketchup shown actually add very few extra calories.

The veggie burger patty plus low-fat cheese amounts to approximately 150 Calories. Add a seeded roll and the total rises to 290 Calories.

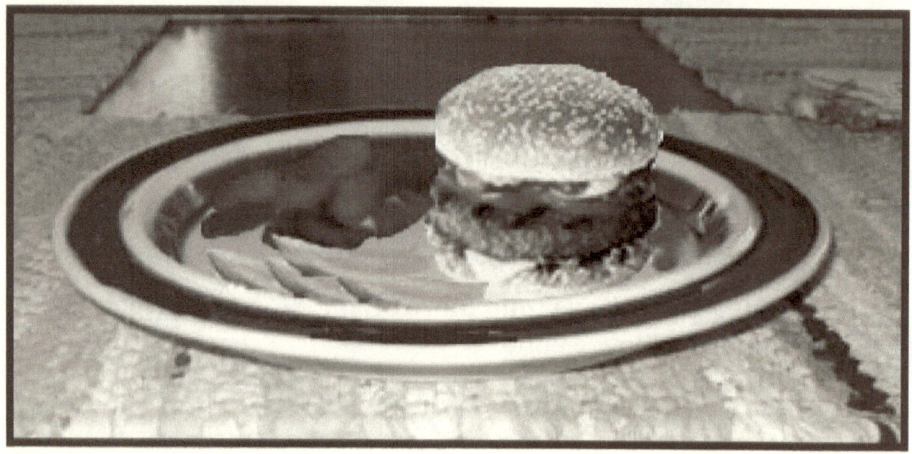

Diet Tip of the Day: **Drink lots of water** – about 8 glasses per day. Add a slice of lemon to make it more interesting. Often, when you think you're hungry, you are just thirsty. So, next time you head for a snack, drink some water first and see if that does it for you.

Day 10 Recipe

Wild Blueberry Pancakes

This recipe makes a relatively low calorie, wholesome batch of delicious wild blueberry-whole grain-buttermilk pancakes.

1 cup whole-grain flour

1 cup buttermilk

1 egg

1 Tbsp vegetable oil

1 tsp baking powder

½ tsp baking soda

Stir ingredients until blended. Add ¾ cup blueberries and gently stir. Using medium heat, preheat a non-stick skillet coated with cooking spray. Pour slightly less than ¼ cup of batter onto skillet per pancake. Cook slowly until bubbles break on surface of pancake. Turn and cook until other side is lightly browned. Makes 8 pancakes.

Pictured below are wild-blueberry pancakes with two slices of turkey bacon.

Serves 4. Each pancake is about 95 Calories

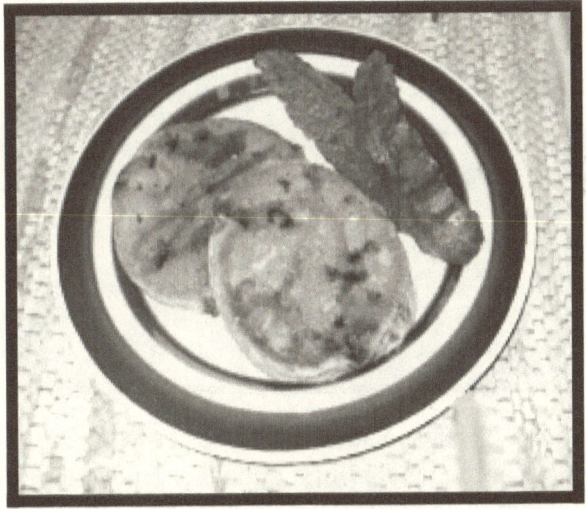

Diet Tip of the Day: A peanut butter sandwich on whole grain bread with a glass of skim milk and an apple makes a nutritious, reasonably low-calorie lunch.

Day 11 Recipe

Artichoke-Bean Salad

1 can (19 oz) white kidney beans
10 artichoke hearts, quartered
⅓ cup chopped oregano
⅓ cup chopped parsley
3 cloves garlic, chopped
1 lemon, juiced
Combine ingredients in medium-size bowl. Stir in ¼ cup Evoo. Salt and black pepper to taste.
Serves 6. Artichoke-bean salad has approximately 190 Calories per serving.
Pictured on the plate below are two grilled chicken sausage links with salsa, steamed green beans and the artichoke-bean salad. Incidentally, this artichoke-bean combination over mixed salad greens served with a whole-grain bread makes a delicious, nutritious and reasonable low-calorie main course.

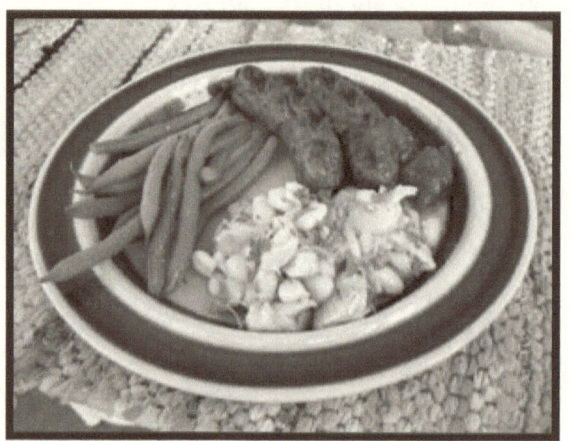

Diet Tip of the Day: Have a small meal before you go to a party. A hardboiled egg, an apple, and a thirst quencher (like water, tea, seltzer, or diet soda) will take the edge off your appetite and make it easier to resist the high-calorie goodies.

Day 12 Recipe
Fish Dinner - Out

No recipe today. No cooking today. Have a fish dinner at your favorite restaurant, but make sure you choose a restaurant where you have a good chance to achieve your calorie goal. For Day 12, your **goal for dinner is a maximum of 595 Calories**. This includes appetizer, soup, main course and dessert.

Tips for Eating Out: The following is almost an exact repeat of advice given for Day 7. First, order simple, such as broiled fish with steamed vegetables and brown rice. Tell the waiter you want no sauce, no gravy, nothing added. Then, knowing your calorie objective, and that fish is about 50 Calories per ounce, most steamed vegetable servings average approximately 50 Calories per cup, and rice is about 100 Calories per ½ cup, decide how much to eat – and take the remainder home. If fresh fruit is not an option, pass on dessert and have the evening snack specified for that day in the diet.

In a restaurant, I recommend you eat the low-calorie items on your plate first. Start with the salad, soup and veggies. By the time you get to the fish and starches you will hopefully be full enough to be content with smaller portions of the higher-calorie choices.

Diet Tip of the Day: Phytonutrients are found in plant foods such as fruits, vegetables, whole grains, dried beans, nuts and seeds. Unlike protein, fat, vitamins and minerals, phytonutrients are not necessary for life, but evidence is growing that phytonutrients have many beneficial qualities.

Day 13 Recipe
Pasta with Marinara Sauce

Prepare the sauce as you did for the Day 6 pizza. But because the pizza sauce is a bit too thick, add ¼ cup of pasta liquid to thin it. (The spiral pasta shape shown below is called Fusilli, and is a favorite because all the ridges really hold the sauce.)

½ pound <u>whole-grain</u> pasta

¼ tsp salt

Prepare the marinara tomato sauce as per Day 6 sauce but dilute it with ¼ cup of pasta liquid. Bring 2 quarts of lightly salted water to a boil. Add pasta and stir occasionally (to keep pasta from sticking to the bottom of the pot). Keep water boiling and cook until pasta are "al dente." (Cooking time is approximately 9 minutes.) Drain pasta, add marinara sauce and serve hot.

<u>Serves 4</u>. One serving is about 225 Calories.

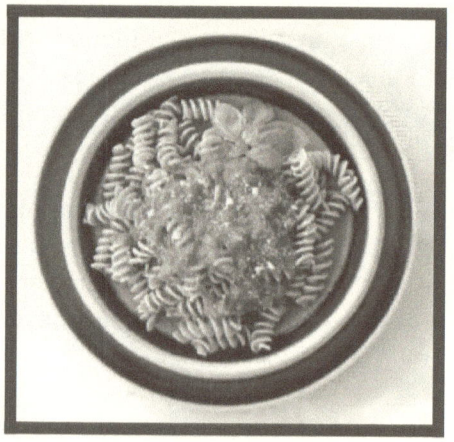

<u>Diet Tip of the Day:</u> **Beware of alcoholic beverages**. Beer has about 13 Calories per ounce, wine 25 Calories per ounce and whiskey 71 Calories per ounce.

Day 14 Recipe
"Oatena" Cereal Mix

Mixing nutritious cereals, hot or cold, is a good way to add variety as well as nutrition to a meal. This recipe features a mix of two whole grain cereals: Oatmeal and Wheatena.

⅓ cup Oatmeal
¼ cup (4 Tbsp) Wheatena
¾ cup water
½ cup skim milk
¼ cup blueberries
10 raisins

Add Oatmeal, Wheatena, raisins and a dash of salt to a microwave-safe cereal bowl. Next add water and stir. Place bowl in microwave, on high power for about 1½ minutes, or until desired consistency is reached. The result is "Oatena," a mix of oatmeal and Wheatena, shown (half eaten) below.

Add skim milk and blueberries and serve hot. Because of the natural sugar in blueberries and raisins, adding sugar is not necessary.

Serves 1. About 310 Calories per serving

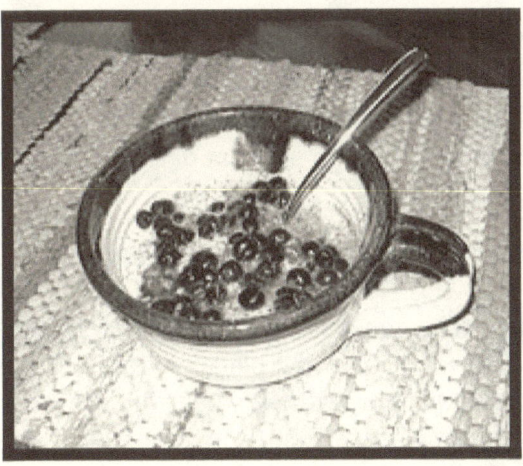

Diet Tip of the Day: Hot or cold cereal topped with fruit, and fat-free milk makes a nutritious, relatively low-calorie meal anytime.

Day 14 Recipe-b
Frozen Chicken Meal

No recipe today. No cooking today. Another day off! Some reasonably good frozen-chicken dinners are:

Poultry	Crustless Chicken Pot Pie	Smart Ones	~~200~~ 190
Poultry	Buffalo Style Chicken	Lean Cuisine	~~200~~ 190
Poultry	Home Style Chicken & Potatoes	Healthy Choice	200
Poultry	Honey Balsamic Chicken	Healthy Choice	210
Poultry	Sesame Stir Fry with Chicken	Lean Cuisine	280
Poultry	Roasted Turkey Breast	Lean Cuisine	~~280~~ 290
Poultry	Apple Cranberry Chicken	Lean Cuisine	280
Poultry	Chicken Fettuccini Alfredo	Healthy Choice	280
Poultry	Grilled Chicken Marinara	Healthy Choice	280
Poultry	Sweet & Spicy Orange Chicken	Healthy Choice	280
Poultry	Chicken Parmesan	Smart Ones	280
Poultry	Turkey Breast with Stuffing	Smart Ones	280

If you choose any of the above you will fall short of the **300 Calories allocated for this Day 14 meal.** In this case, use the remaining 100 or so calories anyway you wish. Splurge on extra dessert or save the calories for the next day.

Please read the important **Frozen-Food Safety Warning** in Appendix B.

<u>Diet Tip of the Day:</u> The **general weight-change rule is "last on first off."** Assume as you gained weight, the first place you noticed it was on your thighs, next your buttocks, then your face. As you lose weight, it generally will come off in the reverse order, first from your face, then your rear and finally your thighs. And there is not much you can do about that. The truth is there is no food, no exercise, no magic belt, and no pill that will cause your body to lose fat in one place rather than another.

Day 15 Recipe
London Broil
1 pound boneless flank steak about ¾" thick, trimmed of fat
1 clove garlic
1 tsp dry oregano
Rub each side of the flank steak with garlic. Season with oregano, salt
and pepper to taste. Prepare a large non-stick skillet over high heat.
Steak should sizzle when placed on hot skillet. Sear steak on one side
for about 5 minutes; then turn and sear other side for about 4 minutes, or
until done to preference. Check the center by making small incision.
Carve into ¼-inch slices.
Serves 4. About 320 Calories per serving (for meat only).

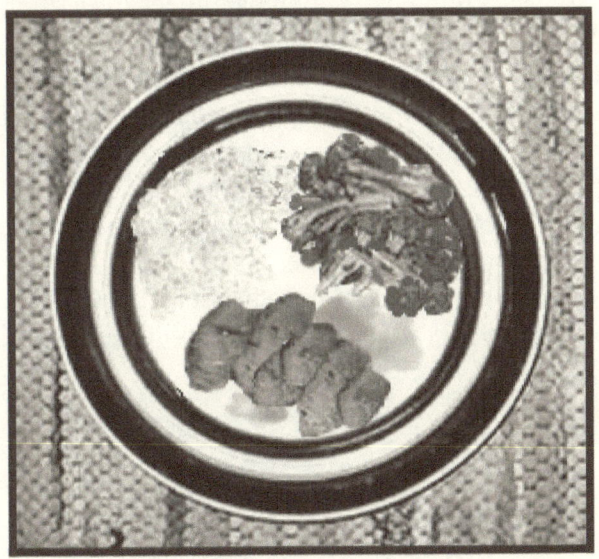

Diet Tip of the Day: **Stay Busy.** Most people will do anything to avoid
work, housework, yard work, exercise, etc. But any kind of work burns
a lot more calories than just sitting! Whatever it is you are avoiding –
just go do it!

Day 16 Recipe

Baked Red Snapper

4 red snapper fillets – 4 oz each (salmon may be substituted)
½ cup white wine
½ cup non-fat yogurt mixed with half as much mustard
½ pound green beans
20 cherry tomatoes
4 tsp olive oil
1 cup wild rice, brown rice and grain berry mix
Prepare rice mix per package directions.

Brown fillets in non-stick pan. Place fillets skin side down in baking dish coated with non-stick spray. Add white wine and cook in oven preheated to 350 °F for about 15 minutes. Spoon pan juices over fillets. Salt and pepper to taste.

Place green beans in skillet. Add ¼-inch of water and cook over medium heat until water boils off. Add cherry tomatoes and olive oil. Stir well and sauté for a few minutes. Season with fresh rosemary and oregano. Salt and pepper to taste.

Plate red snapper fillet and spoon over yogurt-mustard sauce. Add green beans & tomato mix and the wild rice. Serve hot.

Serves 4. One plate consisting of one snapper fillet (215 Calories) with green beans & tomato mix (75 Calories) and wild rice (160 Calories) totals 450 Calories.

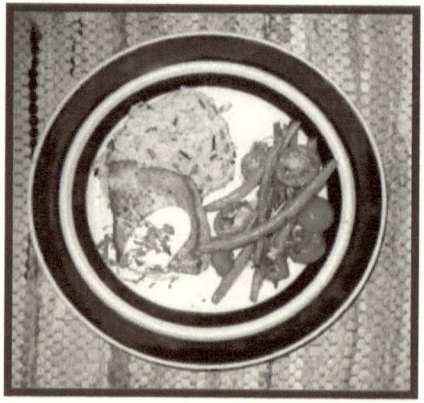

Diet Tip of the Day: **Don't have sweets in your house**. This makes them easier to resist. Out of sight, out of mind!

Day 17 Recipe
Cajun Chicken Salad
This is a perfect after-work, quick, nutritious and delicious dinner.

4 boneless and skinless chicken breasts (about 5 oz each)
1 bottle Cajun spices
8 ounces mixed salad greens
20 cherry tomatoes
12 pitted black olives

Brush chicken breasts lightly with olive oil. Roll breasts in Cajun spices. Brown breasts on non-stick oven-proof skillet. After breasts are brown, put skillet in 350 °F oven for approximately 15 minutes, or until done. Cut breasts into ½-inch slices. (When the breasts are done, the meat should be moist and white with no sign of pink.) Serve hot or keep in an oven or warmer at 200 °F until ready to plate.

Place chicken slices over a bed of mixed salad greens. Add tomatoes, olives and 2 Tbsp of your favorite low-calorie salad dressing.

Serves 4. 330 Calories per serving.

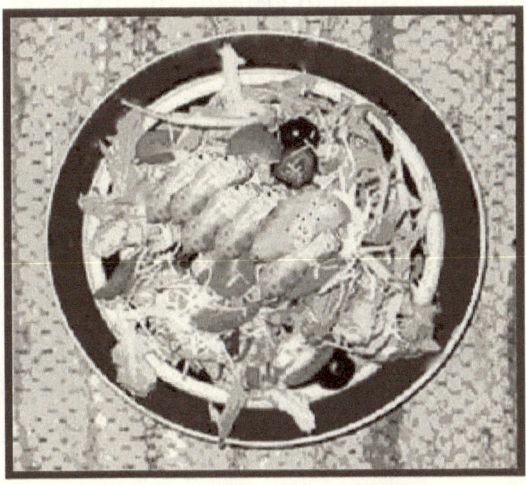

Diet Tip of the Day: Know that **fat-free isn't always your best bet**. Very often sugar is substituted for fat and the calorie total remains the same. Low fat does not necessarily mean low calorie! Rather, look for low-calorie or reduced-calorie products.

Day 18 Recipe

Grilled Swordfish

1¼ pounds swordfish
1 bottle citrus-herb marinade
24 cherry tomatoes
4 medium potatoes
2 cups fresh spinach
1 tsp rosemary & juice of ¼ lemon
2 tsp extra virgin olive oil (Evoo)

Steam spinach with garlic and drizzle with Evoo. Cut up potatoes and place sprinkle with lemon juice, add rosemary, salt and black pepper. Place on grill for about 10 minutes, turning occasionally.

Toss cherry tomatoes in small amount Evoo. Add fresh oregano, salt and black pepper. Place on heavy-duty aluminum foil, seal and grill for about 3 minutes.

Marinade swordfish in citrus-herb vinaigrette. Grill on hot fire for about 5 minutes on one side and 3 minutes on the other, or until done as desired.

Serves 4. One plate consisting of grilled swordfish (250 Calories) with grilled potatoes (100 Calories) and cherry tomatoes (45 Calories) and steamed spinach (50 Calories) totals 445 Calories.

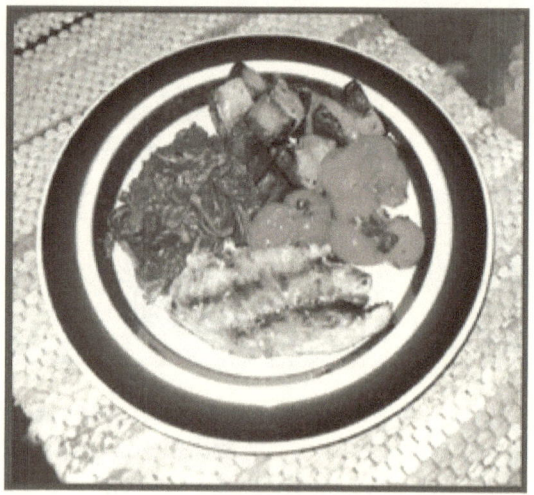

Diet Tip of the Day: Don't be in a hurry to lose weight. Slow weight loss is healthier, is more likely to be permanent, and is easier to sustain over the long haul.

Day 19 Recipe

Chinese Food - Out

No recipe today. No cooking today. Have a Chinese dinner at your favorite restaurant, but make sure you choose a restaurant where you have a reasonable chance to achieve your calorie goal. For today, **your goal for dinner is a maximum of 640 Calories**. This includes any appetizer, soup, main course and any dessert.

Tips for Eating Chinese: You can consume a lot of calories in a Chinese restaurant – if you order carelessly. For example a typical portion of General Tso's chicken is loaded with about 1000 Calories, then add another 200 Calories for a cup of rice.

First rule, order simple. Look for a dish with lots of vegetables, some fish or chicken and brown rice. Tell the waiter you want your food steamed with any sauce on the side. (This is not only a low-calorie way of eating Chinese food but is also the most nutritious way to eat Chinese.)

Then, knowing your 640 Calorie objective, and that chicken and fish are about 50 Calories per ounce, most steamed vegetable servings average approximately 50 Calories per cup, and rice is about 200 Calories per cup, decide how much of the meal you can eat – and take the remainder home. Pass on dessert and have the evening snack specified for that day in the diet. Also see section on **Eating Out** (page 8) for more guidance.

<u>Diet Tip of the Day:</u> Another dilemma for dieters is **judging portion size**. It makes no sense to worry about whether to apportion 70 or 80 Calories per ounce for a cut of lean meat if you have no idea whether the portion you are planning to eat weighs four or ten ounces. To be successful, you must learn to estimate portion sizes with reasonable accuracy.

Day 20 Recipe
Quick Pasta alla Puttanesca
This famous pasta dish originated in Naples. Puttanesca means "ladies of the night." The exact origin of the name is unclear, but one thing is clear: It's delicious! Here is one of many recipe versions.

½ pound spaghetti (whole grain preferred)
20 black pitted olives
1 can (14½ oz) diced tomatoes
½ can (4 oz) tomato sauce
2 Tbsp Evoo
3 cloves of garlic, chopped and 1Tbsp dried minced onion
½ tsp crushed red pepper flakes
1 Tbsp capers drained and rinsed
¼ cup currants

Cook spaghetti according to package directions. Drain and return spaghetti to pot; add a teaspoon Evoo and toss to coat.

Heat 2 tablespoons olive oil in large skillet over medium-high heat. Add red pepper flakes; cook and stir 1 to 2 minutes or until sizzling. Add onion and garlic; cook and stir 1 minute. Finally, add tomatoes with juice, tomato sauce, olives, currants and capers. Cook over medium-high heat, stirring frequently, until sauce is heated through.

Serves 4. About 345 Calories per serving

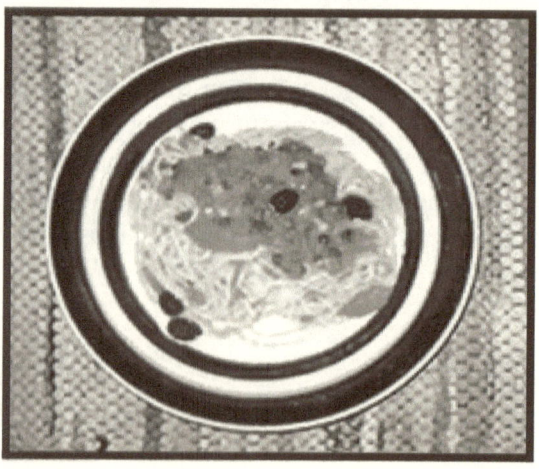

Diet Tip of the Day: Dilute juices, such as apple juice, orange, etc. with water. This cuts the flavor slightly but really reduces calorie content.

Day 21 Recipe
Frozen-Meat Dinner

No recipe today. No cooking today. Another day off! Some reasonably good frozen-meat dinners are:

Meat	Steak Portobella	Lean Cuisine	160
Meat	**Asian Style Beef & Broccoli**	**Smart Ones**	~~160~~ 170
Meat	**Beef Merlot**	**Healthy Choice**	180
Meat	**Home style Beef Pot Roast**	**Smart Ones**	180
Meat	**Salisbury Steak w Mac & Cheese**	**Lean Cuisine**	~~270~~ 290
Pasta	**Pasta with Swedish Meatballs**	**Smart Ones**	~~280~~ 290
Meat	**Classic Meat Loaf**	**Healthy Choice**	300

If you fall short of the **300 Calories allocated for this Day 21 entree**. In this case, use the remaining 100 or so calories anyway you wish. Splurge on extra dessert or save the calories for the next day.

<u>Diet Tip of the Day:</u> A good understanding of nutrition is not only vital for good health but also will help you control your weight over the long term. For example, did you know that foods that are an "excellent source" of a particular nutrient provide 20% or more of the Recommended Daily Value. Whereas, foods that are a "good source" of a nutrient provide between 10 and 20% of the Recommended Daily Value.

Day 22 Recipe

Shrimp & Spinach Salad

2 pounds shrimp in shell
½ pound small green beans, trimmed
½ pound baby spinach leaves
2 Tbsp lemon juice
¼ cup Evoo
2 tsp minced fresh dill
1 Tbsp minced green onion

To make vinaigrette, combine lemon juice, olive oil, dill, salt and pepper to taste and whisk until blended. Stir in minced onion and set aside.

Peel, de-vein and butterfly shrimp. Place shrimp in a bowl and add water to cover. Add 1 teaspoon of salt, and let stand for 10 minutes. Drain, rinse, drain again, and dry. Arrange shrimp in broiling pan without a rack. Brush shrimp with a little vinaigrette and place under preheated broiler, about 3 inches from heat. Broil about 3 to 4 minutes, turning shrimp once, or until both sides turn pink.

Remove shrimp from broiler and add remaining vinaigrette and green beans to the broiling pan. Stir to coat shrimp and beans with vinaigrette. Pour warm vinaigrette over spinach and toss quickly. Plate the spinach and arrange shrimp and green beans on top.

Serves 4. 310 Calories per serving.

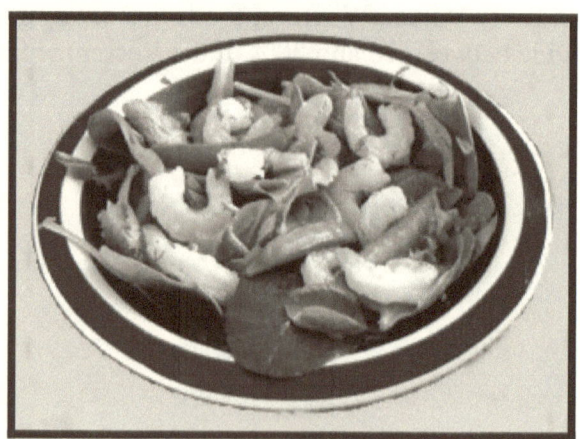

Diet Tip of the Day: After company leaves, have them take some of the leftover food (particularly the dessert) with them – or take the leftovers to work the next day.

Day 23 Recipe
Beans & Greens Salad

⅓ cup chopped oregano
⅓ cup chopped parsley
3 cloves garlic, chopped
1 lemon, juiced
Prepare salad dressing by combining above ingredients and stirring in ¼ cup Evoo. Salt and pepper to taste.
½ pound mesclun mix
¼ pound green beans
1 19 oz can garbanzo beans (chickpeas)
Arrange mesclun mix, garbanzo beans and green beans on a large platter. Drizzle salad dressing over beans and greens.
<u>Serves 4</u>. Approximately 260 Calories per serving.

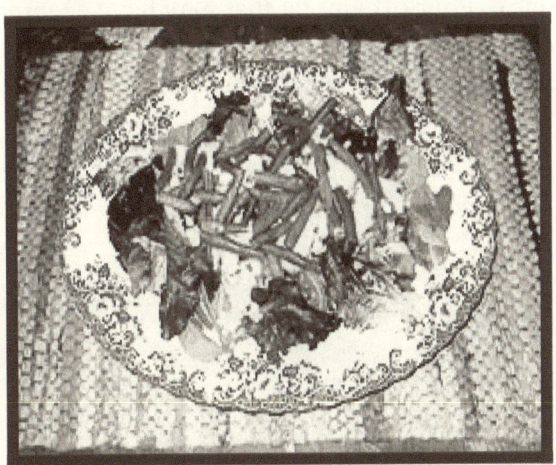

<u>Diet Tip of the Day:</u> Beans are a wonderful food but they are an incomplete protein. If however beans are eaten with a whole-grain bread, the combination forms a complete protein – just as complete and nutritious as meat, poultry, or fish.

Day 24 Recipe

Pan-Broiled Hanger Steak

1¼ pounds hanger steak, well trimmed of fat

¼ cup lime juice

8 small new potatoes, peeled and halved

12 cherry tomatoes, cut in half

Season both sides of steak with salt and pepper and place in sealable plastic bag with lime juice. Refrigerate for about one hour.

Boil potatoes about 10 minutes. Rinse in cold water. Sauté potatoes in small amount of vegetable oil over medium-high heat until brown.

Sauté cherry tomatoes in small amount of olive oil over medium-high heat until skin begins to crack. Season with chopped fresh basil.

Heat a skillet over medium-high heat. Sear hanger steak on one side for about 5 minutes. Turn over and sear other side approximately 5 minutes (for medium done). Pour off any fat that may have accumulated. Carve into ½-inch slices.

Serves 4. About 320 Calories per serving (for the hanger steak only)

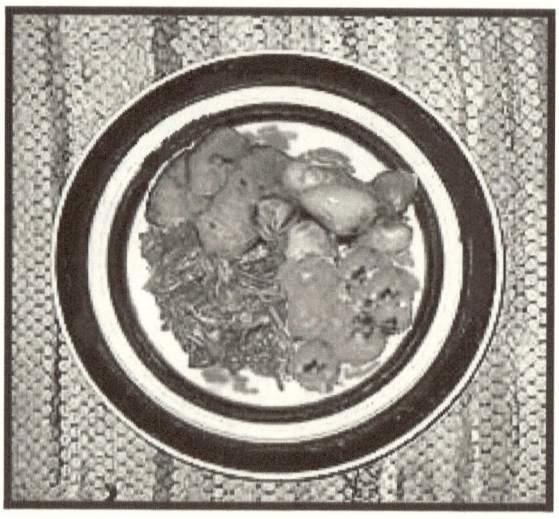

Diet Tip of the Day: If you find yourself at a party, don't stand near the food! Be aware of the temptation. Make the effort, and you'll find you eat less.

Day 25 Recipe
Grilled Scallops and Polenta

1 pound sea scallops
¾ cup polenta cornmeal
¾ cup skim milk
1 medium Portobello mushroom
½ pound green beans
¼ cup chopped red onion
16 asparagus spear
1 tsp Evoo

Bring 1½ cups of water and skim milk to rapid boil. Add salt to taste and slowly add polenta while stirring. Reduce heat. Continue stirring until desired consistency is reached. Pour polenta into lightly greased pan. After polenta has cooled cover and refrigerate. Cut chilled polenta into 4 pieces. Grill on medium-hot fire – about two minutes on each side.

Brush Portobello mushroom and asparagus spear with Evoo and place on grill for about 3 minutes on each side.

Grill scallops on medium-hot fire. Turn after two minutes or when first side turns opaque. Grill until second side turns opaque – about another 2 minutes. Don't overcook but test a scallop by cutting to make sure it's cooked through. Salt and pepper to taste.

<u>Serves 4</u>. The food on the plate pictured below totals 380 Calories.

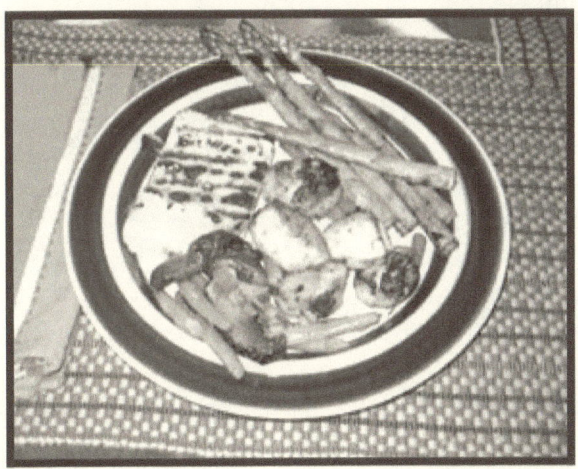

<u>Diet Tip of the Day:</u> To have better control of what you eat **bring your lunch to work**.

APPENDIX A
Calories in Foods

Zero Calorie Foods
Beverages
Coffee without added sugar, cream, or milk
Tea without added sugar, cream, or milk
Carbonated beverages, artificially sweetened
Diet soda
Seltzer water, Sparkling water
Seasoning Agents
Celery seasoning*, Celery salt
Chives seasoning*
Cinnamon
Curry powder
Dill, Garlic*
Herbs, Horseradish*
Lemon juice, sections, or slices*
Lime juice, sections, or slices*
Mint
Monosodium glutamate
Mustard, Onion salt
Onion seasoning*
Paprika, Parsley*
Pepper, all varieties
Peppers, garden, red or green, as seasoning*
Pimiento as seasoning*
Salt, Salt substitutes
Sauces (Worcestershire, A-1, Tabasco
Spices
Vinegar, cider, or wine
Relishes
Bread and butter pickles*
Cucumber & Dill pickles*
India relish*
Pickled onion*
Sour pickles*

Soups
Bouillon
Clear soups without fat
Consommé*
Jellied clear soups*
Jellied consommé*
Tomato bouillon*
Jellied madrilène*
Others
Gelatin, unsweetened*
Sugar Substitutes
Saccharin, Aspartame
* These items contain a few calories, but the calorie counts are negligible when they are used as seasoning, a relish or a thickening agent.

Calories in Beverages
Soda such as Colas, 7-Up (8 oz) ..100 Calories
Beer & ale (12 oz) ....175 Calories
Dry wines (4 oz) ....100 Calories
Whisky (jigger) ....125 Calories
Cocktail (12 oz) .... 150 Calories

Calories in Meat, Poultry & Fish
The calories in meat, poultry and fish largely depend on fat content, both visible and invisible. These foods are divided into three groups: lean, moderately fat, and fat. The calorie values below apply to cooked products after visible fat has been removed. Note, when dieting chose only from the lean and moderately fat groups.
<u>Very Lean Shellfish</u> (25 Cal/Oz)
Clams, Crabmeat
Lobster, Mussels
Oysters, Scallops
Shrimp
<u>Lean Meats & Poultry</u> (50 Cal/Oz) – trim fat
Chicken
Dried or chipped beef
Game, Heart
Kidney, Liver
Turkey bacon (35 Cal/slice)

Turkey, Veal
Lean Fish **(50 Cal/Oz)**
Abalone, Bluefish
Bonito, Butterfish
Cod, Eels, raw
Flounder, Haddock
Halibut, Herring, raw
Ocean perch
Pike, lake, Pollack
Salmon, fresh or canned
Shad, Shad roe
Sturgeon
Swordfish, Tilefish
Tuna, fresh/canned in water (35 Cal/Oz)
Weakfish, Whitefish
Moderately Fatty Meats **(75 Cal/Oz)** – trim fat
Beef, Bologna
Ham, Hot dogs
Lamb, Pork
Tongue
Moderately Fat Fish **(75 Cal/Oz)**
Bass, average
Herring, pickled
Mackerel, Sardines
Trout, brook
Tuna, canned in oil
Fatty Meats, Poultry & Fish **(90 Cal/Oz)** – trim fat
Eel, smoked
Duck, Goose
Luncheon meats
Sweetmeats
Trout, lake

Calories in Vegetables
Any vegetable may be substituted for any other fruit or vegetable with the same calorie count.
25 Calories per cup
Artichoke (1 medium)

Asparagus (6 spears)
Beans (snap, green, wax)
Cabbage, Cauliflower
Celery, Chard
Cucumber, Endive
Escarole, Lettuce
Mushrooms, Parsley
Peppers, Pickles
Pimentos, Radishes
Scallions
Squash (summer)
Tomato (1 medium)
Tomato juice, Watercress

50 Calories per cup

Bean sprouts, Kohlrabi
Beet greens, Mustard greens
Beets, Broccoli
Brussels sprouts
Carrots, Eggplant
Fennel, Kale
Okra, Rutabagas
Sauerkraut
Spinach
Turnip greens, Turnips

100 Calories per cup

Collards
Dandelion greens
Onion (1 medium)
Parsnips
Potato (1 medium)
Pumpkin, Rice (100 Cal per ½ cup)
Leeks, Squash (winter)

150 Calories per cup

Beans, lima
Corn, Peas
Sweet potato (1 medium)

Calories in Fruit

Any fruit may be substituted for any other fruit or vegetable with the same calorie count.

50 Calories per cup (or as indicated)
Apricots (raw, 3)
Cantaloupe (½ medium)
Cranberries, Currants
Fruit salad (raw or water packed)
Gooseberries
Honeydew melon
Lemon or Lime (2 medium)
Lemon or Lime juice
Nectarines (2 small)
Plums (2), Rhubarb
Strawberries
Tangerines (2 small)
Watermelon

75 Calories
Apple (1 medium)
Grapefruit (½ medium)
Orange (1 medium)

100 Cal/cup (or as indicated)
Applesauce, Apricot
Banana (1 medium)
Blackberries
Blueberries
Cherries
Dates (4 raw or dried)
Grapefruit (sections or juice)
Prunes (4 medium)
Figs (3 small), Grapes
Loganberries
Orange (sections or juice)
Papayas
Peaches (raw or canned)
Pears (raw or canned)
Pineapple (raw or juice)
Raspberries

150 Calories per cup
Apple juice, Mango

Grape juice
Persimmons, Guava
Plums (raw or canned)
Prune juice (200 Calories per cup)
Raisins (500 Calories per cup)

Calories in Dairy Products
Whole milk 150 Cal/cup
Skim milk 80 Cal/cup
Yogurt - Whole milk - plain (180 Cal/cup)
Yogurt - Fat-free – plain (90 Cal/cup)
Yogurt – Fat-free - frozen choc (240 Cal/cup)
Cottage cheese - whole milk (220 Cal/cup)
Cottage cheese - fat free (160 Cal/cup)
All other cheese 100 Cal/Oz
Ice cream:
Whole milk (300 Cal/cup)
Light (240 Cal/cup)
Fat free (220 Cal/cup)
Sherbet (250 Cal/cup)
Egg medium (80 Calories)

Bread and Cereals
Bagels (3½" dia) 200 Cal
Biscuits (2" dia) 100.Cal
Cereal Cooked (½ cup) 75 Cal
Cereal Dry (¾ cup) 100 Cal
Corn bread (2" square) 150 Cal
Melba toast (1 piece) 25 Cal
Most bread (1 slice) 65 Cal
Rolls (average) 100 Cal
Ry-Crisp (1 piece) 25 Cal
Crackers, Cookies & Cake
Graham (1 whole cracker) . 100 Cal
Angel food (2 oz) .... 175 Cal

Calories in Oils and Nuts
Butter 50 Calories per pat (16 pats per ¼ lb)
Nuts 100 Calories per handful
Peanut butter 100 Cal/Tbsp

Salad dressings 75 Cal/Tbsp
Vegetable Oils 125 Cal/Tbsp

APPENDIX B
Frozen Food Safety

Increasingly, food giants like ConAgra, Nestlé and others that supply Americans with processed foods concede that they cannot ensure the safety of their food products. Frozen foods pose a particularly serious safety problem because unsuspecting consumers buy frozen foods for their convenience and incorrectly believe that cooking frozen foods is a matter of taste – not safety.

Still the food industry says that extensive outbreaks of food-borne illness are rare, even though it is well-known that most of the millions of cases of food-borne illness every year go unreported or are not traced to the source. For example, each year approximately 40,000 cases of salmonella poisoning are reported in the United States – but perhaps as many as one million cases go unreported. (Salmonella is a type of bacteria most often found in poultry, eggs, unprocessed milk, meat and water.) Recently salmonella pathogens in some frozen meals have sickened thousands of people.

How could this happen? First, the supply chain for ingredients in processed foods – from flour to fruits and vegetables to flavorings – is becoming more complex and global in the drive to keep food costs down. As a result, government and industry officials concede that almost every food ingredient is now a potential carrier of pathogens. A further complication is that a large number of food companies subcontract processing work to save money and don't require suppliers to test for pathogens. In fact, companies often don't even know who is supplying their ingredients.

In addition, many frozen-food manufacturers have stopped cooking their products at high temperatures, a tactic they call the "kill step," which is intended to eliminate any lingering microbes. Frequently this process step turns some of the frozen food ingredients into mush. So, instead the "kill step" has been shifted to consumers. For example, ConAgra has added food safety instructions to its frozen meals, including the Healthy Choice brand. A typical "frozen-food safety" instruction offers this guidance: "Internal temperature needs to reach 165°F as measured by a food thermometer in several spots."

Moreover, General Mills, now advises consumers to avoid microwaves altogether and cook their frozen pizzas only in a conventional oven.

Bottom line: To be safe, always cook frozen foods so that the internal temperature reaches 165°F as measured by a good food thermometer.

APPENDIX C
Soup Selections

When the Daily Meal Plan menu specifies soup have only one serving (8 ounces) unless stated otherwise. Note that the listed soups were available in most supermarkets as of 07/24/2020.   *These are canned soup selections.

Soup Description	Calories
Healthy Choice Chicken with Rice	90
Campbell's Tomato	100
Healthy Choice Country Vegetable	100
Progresso Minestrone*	110
Progresso Chickarina*	110
Progresso Italian-Style Wedding*	120
Campbell's Home-Style Light Chicken Corn Chowder*	120
Campbell's Home-Style Chicken Noodle	130
Campbell's Home-Style Butter Nut Squash*	130
Campbell's Healthy Request Vegetable Beef	140
Progresso Lentil*	140
Progresso Green Split Pea*	150
Campbell's Slow Kettle New England Clam Chowder	160
Progresso Macaroni and Bean*	160
Progresso New England Clam Chowder*	170
Progresso Lasagna-Style*	170
Progresso Broccoli Cheese with Bacon*	180
Also may have 2 servings of a 90 Cal soup	180
Campbell's Chunky Classic Chicken Noodle	190
Amy's Rustic Italian Vegetable*	190
Campbell's Chunky Beef n Cheese*	200
Amy's French Country Vegetable*	210
Campbell's Chunky Sirloin Burger + Vegetables	220
Enjoy two servings of a 110 or 120 Calorie soup	230
Enjoy two servings of a 120 Calorie soup	240

NoPaperPress eBooks and Paperbacks

100-Day Super Diet-1200 Calorie*
100-Day Super Diet-1500 Calorie*
100-Day No-Cooking Diet-1200 Cal*
100-Day No-Cooking Diet-1500 Cal*
90-Day Smart Diet-1200 Calorie*
90-Day Smart Diet-1500 Calorie*
90-Day No-Cooking Diet - 1200 Cal*
90-Day No-Cooking Diet - 1500 Cal*
90-Day Perfect Diet - 1200 Calorie*
90-Day Perfect Diet - 1500 Calorie*
60-Day Perfect Diet-1200 Calorie*
60-Day Perfect Diet-1500 Calorie*
50-Day Flex Diet-1200 Calorie*
50-Day Flex Diet-1500 Calorie*
30-Day Quick Diet - for Women*
30-Day Quick Diet - for Men*
30-Day No-Cooking Diet*
30-Day Diet for Women - Metric*
30-Day Diet for Men - Metric*
25 Day Easy Diet-1200 Calorie*
25 Day Easy Diet-1500 Calorie*
25-Day No-Cooking Diet
10-Day Express Diet
10-Day No-Cooking Diet*
7-Day Diet for Women*
7-Day Diet for Men*
7-Day No-Cooking Diets*
90-Day Gluten-Free Diet-1200 Cal*
90-Day Gluten-Free Diet-1500 Cal*
30-Day Gluten-Free Quick Diet*
30-Day Gluten-Free No-Cooking Diet*
7-Day Diet for Women - Metric*
7-Day Diet for Men - Metric
7-Day Gluten-Free Express Diet*
7-Day Gluten-Free No-Cooking Diet*
90-Day Vegetarian Diet-1200 Calorie*
90-Day Vegetarian Diet-1500 Calorie*
30-Day Vegetarian Diet*
7-Day Vegetarian Diet*
Weight Loss for Women*
Weight Loss for Women - Metric
Weight Loss for Women - UK
Weight Loss for Men*
Maximum Weight Loss - 1200 Cal*
Maximum Weight Loss - 1500 Cal*

Weight Loss for Men - Metric*
Maximum Weight Loss- 1200 Calorie*
Maximum Weight Loss- 1500 Calorie*
Weight Control - U.S. Edition
Weight Control - Metric. Edition
Professional Weight Control Women - U.S.
Professional Weight Control Women - Metric
Professional Weight Control Men - U.S.
Professional Weight Control Men - Metric
Weight Maintenance - U.S. Edition*
Weight Maintenance - Metric. Edition*
Weight Maintenance - UK Edition
Weight Loss for Senior Men*
Weight Loss for Senior Women*
Eat Smart - U.S. Edition*
Eat Smart - Metric Edition
30-Day Mediterranean Diet
Exercise Smart - U.S. Edition*
Exercise Smart - Metric Edition
Exercise Smart - UK Edition*
Total Fitness - U.S. Edition
Total Fitness - Metric Edition
Total Fitness - UK Edition
Total Fitness for Women-U.S. Edition*
Total Fitness for Women - Metric
Total Fitness for Women - UK Edition
Total Fitness for Men - U.S. Edition*
Total Fitness for Men- Metric Edition*
Total Fitness for Men - UK Edition
Senior Fitness - U.S. Edition*
Senior Fitness - Metric Edition*
Senior Fitness - UK Edition*
Computer Diet - U.S. Edition*
Computer Diet - Metric Edition*
Reliable Weight Loss - U.S. Edition
101 Weight Loss Tips*
101 Healthy Eating Tips*
101 Lifelong Fitness Tips*
101 Weight Maintenance Tips
101 Weight Loss Recipes
101 Gluten-Free Weight Loss Recipes
101 Vegetarian Weight Loss Recipes*
30-Day Mediterranean Diet*
90-Day Mediterranean Diet - 1200 Cal*
90-Day Mediterranean Diet - 1500 Cal*

* These titles are available as both ebooks and paperbacks. Our ebooks are sold by Amazon, Apple, Google, Barnes & Noble and Kobo, but our paperbacks are only sold by Amazon.

Disclaimer

This book offers general meal planning, nutrition and weight control information. It is not a medical manual and the author does not claim to be medically qualified. The material in this book is not intended to be a substitute for medical counseling. Everyone should have a medical checkup before beginning a weight loss program. Moreover, the physician conducting the medical exam should be made aware of and should approve the specific weight control program planned. Additionally, while the author and publisher have made every effort to ensure the accuracy of the information in this book, they make no representations or warranties regarding its accuracy or completeness. Further, neither the author nor publisher assume liability for any medical problems that might result from applying the methods in this book, or for any loss of profit, or any other commercial damages, including but not limited to special, incidental, consequential or other damages, and any such liability is hereby expressly disclaimed.